Yoga
against Spinal Pain

by
Pandit Shiv Sharma

Photographs by
Jitendra Arya

GEORGE G. HARRAP & CO. LTD
London   Toronto   Wellington   Sydney

To my wife and daughters
HEM, SHARAT, and HEMANT
who inspired me to resort to writing for self expression
(having never given me a chance to speak during a conversation)
I dedicate this book with affection and warmth

First published in Great Britain 1971
by GEORGE G. HARRAP *&* CO. LTD
182–184 High Holborn, London WC1V 7AX
© *Shiv Sharma* 1971

ISBN 0 245 50629 2

*Set in Monotype Times and printed by photo-lithography
at the Pitman Press, Bath*

Made in Great Britain

ACKNOWLEDGMENTS

I am grateful to:

Dr Kailash Sharma, for reading through the manuscript and making very valuable changes and corrections;

Mr Vijaypat Singhania, the noted industrialist, for placing at my disposal his beautiful suburban villa, Kamla Cottage, on the Juhu Beach, and the Photographic Department of the J.K. Industries for the production of some of the photographs for this book;

Shri Yogendra, the eminent Yogi-savant, and Shri Jayadeva, his distinguished son and disciple, for their unreserved help and guidance;

Shri B. K. S. Iyengar of Poona, the renowned Yogi, from whom I took my first lessons in Yoga;

Yogi Shri Umesh Chandra, who offered me the valuable co-operation of his brilliant son and disciple, Dr N. U. Joshi;

Dr N. U. Joshi, the handsome Yogi, whose photographs appear in this book;

Miss Sophy Kelly, Principal, Hill Grange School, Bombay, who introduced me to the young lady whose photographs adorn the pages of this book;

Miss Orna Herman, who, in spite of being a total stranger to Yoga, and having been brought into the picture to give the Western readers a feeling of self-identification, in view of the mistakes she was expected to make in trying the Yogic postures, sprang a pleasant surprise on all concerned by performing almost all the Asanas, with only two or three exceptions, to perfection;

Dr D. V. Bharati, Editor, *Dharma-yuga*, for kindly arranging the line drawings;

Mr and Mrs Herman, for the exceptional respect they showed for this book by permitting their daughter, Miss Herman, to pose for these photographs;

Mr Vijay Sadanah, the debonair executive of Goel Cine Corporation, for his courtesy and efficiency in cheerfully organizing instantaneous set-ups for photography at annoyingly short notice;

Mr Jitendra Arya, for all the plates in this book, with the exception of Plates 15, 29 (Pose 2), and 31 (Yogi) which are by Mr R. R. Bharadwaj; my thanks to both these eminent photo-artists for their excellent photography;

Mr R. M. Sharma, for his efficiency in looking after the mobility and convenience of all participants in the production of the photographs;

Mr Ligorio Rodrigues, for proving the most non-exasperating, cheerful, and efficient stenographer I ever worked with so far;

The Government of India, for their kindly according me permission to draw on their publication *Yogic Therapy*, by Kuvalayanand and Vinekar.

Cover photographs by Jitendra Arya and R. R. Bharadwaj.

CONTENTS

THE ASANAS

INTRODUCTION

You and I

In ancient India knowledge was the gift of the teacher to his pupil. Knowledge was not sold and teaching was not a business. Rather it was a sacred act of blessing the receiver. The Guru (religious teacher) expected nothing from his pupil but that he should earnestly wish to learn and that he should apply himself to his studies without lapses or laziness. The teacher and the pupil— and the author and the reader—had a deep emotional relationship in the Orient. The teacher was greatly concerned for his pupil, and was in turn regarded with deep and intense affection by him. The only aspect of selfishness traceable in the mental attitude of the teacher was his desire for sincere reverence on the part of his pupil. In return he wanted the pupil to excel even himself—this was the teacher's only reward.

It is my hope that the relationship between myself and my readers shall be similar to that of the teacher and pupil of ancient India. This book may be short, but that is not an indication, I hope, of its value. If, after going through these pages, you can find and develop a firm basis for abiding happiness and enjoyment of life, relaxation and tranquillity, fitness and longevity; if it imparts a spiritual yet radiant outlook on life, then I will be satisfied and rewarded.

It is within your power to offer me that fulfilment. You can do it by going through the pages of this book carefully and following the instructions earnestly and faithfully. You will not find the text difficult to follow. Whilst I have had to use a few technical terms, both medical and Yogic, these are carefully explained wherever they occur.

What Yoga Offers

Any one can suffer physical pain. Pain can afflict the ignorant and the clever, the poor and the rich, the male and the female, the young and the old, the strong and the weak. Everybody needs the

9

guidance contained in this book. The amount of benefit you reap will depend only on your own determination and your ability to overcome the inertia which may hamper you in beginning the practices described. The way is open to all, the obstacles are not insurmountable, and relief from pain is easily within your reach.

Once you have experienced a sense of mental and physical well-being, enabling you to enjoy life to the full, you will need no further encouragement to stick to a health-giving routine. By a judicious and scientific mobilization of the extensive and un-exploited inner resources of your own body, and with no external aids and no drugs whatsoever, you can be free of racking pain and tension. This is what Yoga offers you. As you will find out for yourself, it is no exaggerated claim.

It should be borne in mind that steadiness and strength of mind are closely linked with the fitness of the body. In no other technique is the interdependence of the mind and body demonstrated so effectively as in the practice of Yoga. As a liberator of the body and the mind of man, Yoga is unparalleled.

The Rationale of Yoga

Although your main object in studying this book is to learn the practices which can relieve you of your pains, rigidities, and tensions and to acquire a natural tranquillity and steadiness of the mind through your knowledge and practice of Yoga, I feel sure that many of you will want to know how the mechanism works which achieves this end. Those of you who consider a study of the theoretical aspects of the Yogic approach to health and disease unnecessary and accept the practical guidance as adequate for your needs are welcome to skip over this section of the book.

In the explanation which follows I shall not be able to avoid some technical words which are necessary to give a clear idea of how physical posture influences mental attitude.

For those wishing to understand the mechanism of the practice of Yoga I must answer the significant question, "How can a few twists and turns of the body change the attitudes of the mind for the better?"

Most of you are aware of the simple fact that the nervous system is roughly divided into sensory and motor components. The sensory nerves are those which carry impulses to the brain, and

10

the motor nerves carry impulses from the brain back to the muscles and various organs. The sensory system is served by two types of receptors, the exteroceptive and the interoceptive. Exteroceptors, as the name implies, receive stimuli from the world around us and are present in the eyes, ears, nose, mouth, skin, and mucous membranes. With their help we recognize touch, temperature, taste, smell, and pain, and are able to see and hear.

The interoceptors are situated in the deeper strata—such as muscles, tendons, joints, viscera (various organs of the body), blood vessels, the internal ear, etc. They are constantly supplying the lower brain centres with information on the positions of various parts of the body relative to each other, and on the state of tension of various muscles and tendons.

The neuromuscular or motor system has a dual nature—phasic and tonic. Of these two, the phasic component is more obvious, and more easily observable. The movements of the eyeballs, the swinging of the arms, or the movement of the legs when walking are all phasic reactions. But it is the tonic reaction which not only forms the background for phasic reaction, but also sustains or inhibits it. The interoceptive-tonic mechanism does not impinge on the conscious. In general, the exteroceptive impulses excite the phasic reactions (which are passing) while the interoceptive impulses regulate the tonic reactions. It is important to remember that while the phasic movement is momentary, involving a group of muscles, the interoceptive-tonic mechanism is continuous and diffuse and provides at all times the means by which phasic movements are possible.

But muscle tone is only a part of a much bigger whole. The whole integrated phenomenon in modern physiological psychology is called the 'postural substrate'. The word 'postural' here denotes an all-inclusive (neuro-musculo-glandular) background which influences every action of our body no matter how trivial or momentary.

The rôle of visceral tension and glandular secretion is as yet far from clear. We do know, however, that the sum total of all these specific tensions provides the organism with a continuous and, in ideal circumstances, homogeneous background which influences all movement and reactions of the body, both external and internal.

It is obvious that the 'postural substrate' in a normal organism

11

is and has to be in a continuously dynamic and fluid state, varying with the demand made on the body or mind, in order to provide an ideal background for any action contemplated. What is not so obvious is that the elasticity of this extremely malleable 'substrate' can, under conditions of stress and disease, be strained to the limit. This can lead to disintegration.

Yoga teaches that by attacking the abnormal postural substrate and reconditioning it to its previous adaptable and dynamic state, modification of the emotional state can be obtained, leading to a state of mental tranquillity.

Actually, since most of the tensions causing such a physico-psychological derangement are of long standing, they of necessity require a long time for a cure. This is eventually accomplished by 'Dhyana' or meditation at a spiritual level, but the immediate attack is started at a physical level by 'Asanas' (Yogic postures) and 'Pranayama' (Life-Breath Culture).

Asanas (Yogic Postures) and Backache
'Oiling' the Psychosomatic Machine

Asanas, literally translated, means 'postures'. But they are more than that, as you will see when you find that Yoga always involves the mind with the body. The detailed how and why of all Asanas are beyond the scope of this book. *Gheranda Samhita*, an ancient compendium, refers to literally thousands of Asanas or Yogic postures!

However, it is necessary to review and further explain a few salient points regarding these postures. I have already explained how the muscle tone is controlled and modified by the interplay of sensory impulses from various parts of the body and the higher brain centres; how the normally flexible, supple, and elastic muscle can be distorted and made rigid by a disturbed psyche resulting in a continuous lack of equilibrium in body and mind, and how Yoga can help restore this.

This does not imply that the practice of Yoga is meant exclusively for the benefit of the psychologically unbalanced. While, un-doubtedly, Yoga is effective for people in this condition, we are here concerned with that aspect of it which, by 'oiling' the various parts of the body and mind, ensures a smooth running and efficient working of the psychosomatic machine.

12

Man has paid the price of acquiring an erect posture in the form of an increased predisposition to backache. A sedentary life and the resultant increase in obesity causes a laxity of the body musculature, in particular the supporting part, which has made backache as common a condition as the common cold.

Whether you are a man or a woman, you will be able to judge for yourself the tremendous benefit to be got from Yoga with relatively little effort.

The most important point you have to realize before starting the practice of Yoga is that the Asanas are not just simple exercises but sustained, scientific patterns of posture. No jerky movements are involved and even in some dynamic Asanas, the movement has to be of a slow, spontaneous, uniform nature. The neuro-muscular system is so composed that for every group of muscles that go into contraction, another group undergoes relaxation. In tension states this reciprocal innervation becomes defective. Asanas, by their very nature, reorganize and recondition the system to bring about physiological harmony between the two.

According to the classics, the object of the Asanas is to provide stability and well-being. To achieve this it is necessary that the Asana be performed without any conscious control so that while the body is in a particular pose, the mind is free for contemplation. This is not easy. I will elucidate it further.

If you see a baby trying to take his first steps, you find that his whole being is concentrated in the performance of the action of putting one foot in front of the other. Even a momentary break in concentration causes him to topple and clutch for the nearest support. Now, compare this with the effortless ease with which you yourself walk or stand. It does not require any conscious thought or concentration, and you can indulge in conversation or any other activity without the danger of falling to the ground. It is this sort of conditioning that your system must undergo before you become proficient in the performance of the Asanas.

At first you will have to make a deliberate effort. But gradually, with continuous practice, your body will respond and develop a suppleness and a freedom of movement you never thought possible. Of course, there are people who cannot manage a perfect 'textbook' posture. Let them perform the Asanas imperfectly; they will derive considerable benefit from their practice. There is no

13

need to be disheartened if you cannot put yourself through the same contortions as your Yogic teacher. As long as the effort is made consistently and the maximum possible mobility achieved, Yogic benefits will prove of immense value. At no stage should you strain beyond the sensation of a slight (if mildly pleasurable) pain. Too vigorous an effort may result in harm and negation of the good that would have been done.

Pranayama—The Yogic Breath Culture
Pulmonary Feeder and Vacuum Cleaner

You can overload your stomach with highly seasoned food and harm your health. You cannot overload your lungs with the oxygen-laden fresh air. The more oxygen you breathe into your lungs, the more benefits you reap. There is a natural limit to your intake of breath which automatically protects you against an excess. There is no limiting mechanism to prevent excesses in eating or drinking.

The air you breathe is more essential to life than the food you eat. Without food you can live for days and weeks, perhaps months. But, without air, life ceases within a few minutes, if not seconds. Therefore, nobody discusses health these days without extolling the virtues of deep breathing.

Breathing, like all other vital functions of the body, is regulated and controlled at a subconscious level. We become conscious of it only when the process becomes painful due to disease of the lung, pleura, or chest wall, or is affected by disease of other organs. The fact that most of the time respiration is adjusted to the needs of the body does not necessarily imply that it is being carried out with the maximum of efficiency. The modern man who is not getting enough exercise, is slightly overweight, lacks proper muscle tone, and has a faulty posture, in all probability has a faulty respiration and is in consequence a candidate for diseases of the respiratory tract and for a general lowering of efficiency, both physical and mental.

Let us first define respiration. In layman's terms it is the means whereby oxygen is taken into the body (inspiration) and carbon dioxide—a product of the various oxidizing processes going on in the body—is given out (expiration). No cell in the human body can live without oxygen. Since most of these oxidizing processes

14

are carried out at a subcellular level, it is the cell—the basic unit of our body structure—that suffers most from lack of oxygen. Since the dependence of cells on oxygen varies with the degree of their specialization it is the nervous system which is first and most acutely affected, before the lack becomes manifest in other parts of the body.

I mentioned earlier the type of persons more likely to have faulty respiratory control—*i.e.*, the obese and those with poor posture and muscle tone. The obese are handicapped by the poor excursion of the diaphragm, as are those suffering from poor posture and muscle tone. The contraction of the diaphragm along with the muscles of the chest wall increases the volume of the chest cavity to allow for the full expansion of the lungs and entry of the air. It is obvious that the breathing of a person suffering from faulty posture will automatically improve on doing exercises that help remedy the defect just as improvement in the breathing technique will improve, to a degree, the posture and muscle tone. But it must be remembered that these breathing and postural exercises must supplement each other. To get the maximum benefit both must be practised simultaneously.

Without going into the physiology of respiration, which is a highly technical subject and beyond the scope of this book, the process of breathing may be described as follows: a deep breath aerates all parts of the lungs; by creating a negative intra-thoracic pressure it acts as a suction pump and draws in more blood from the venous side for circulation by the heart. Because of the increased lung capacity, more blood is accommodated and because this blood is in contact with the ventilated areas of the lung, a more thorough exchange of gases takes place. Proper oxygenation of the blood ensures a good supply of this essential commodity to the body tissues. A deep expiration collapses the lungs, expelling the maximum amount of carbon dioxide. Since the next inspiration starts with the lungs maximally collapsed it is automatically deeper, thereby initiating a cycle that ensures the maximum efficiency of the cardio-respiratory unit.

Few modern scientists have any idea of the method of deep breathing prescribed by Yoga. Generally, deep breathing means merely breathing deeply—*i.e.*, deep inhalations followed by exhalations to match. This deep breathing differs from ordinary

15

breathing only in the larger volume of air inhaled and exhaled. It is certainly more advantageous to the system than the average normal breathing, but the Yogic breathing is a further improvement on deep breathing.

One deep breath is a two-unit breath consisting of one inhalation and one exhalation. But a single Yogic (Pranayamic) breath consists of four units:

1. Puruka (literally, that which fills—*i.e.*, inhalation),
2. Kumbhaka (literally, a steady state of full distension of the lungs),
3. Rechaka (literally, that which expels—*i.e.*, exhalation), and
4. Shunyaka (literally, a state of void).

The process is easy to follow. Firstly, a slow and deep breath expands the lungs, bringing the maximum supply of oxygen-laden air to the air spaces. The second stage consists of holding the breath, thereby holding the air spaces in a state of expansion much longer than usual. This pause covers an interval at least twice as long as the time taken by the preceding inhalation. The exhalation also has to be slow and deep to bring about the maximum contraction of the air spaces, so that the maximal outgoing breath, with its carbon dioxide content, is squeezed out of the lungs. The fourth and the final stage is the maintenance of the state of maximum void in the air spaces achieved by the long deep exhalation. Keeping the air out for a brief period is as important in Yogic breathing as the holding of breath after a deep inhalation.

Different schools of Yoga prescribe different periods for four-unit breathing in practice. The ratio, according to the majority view, between different durations of the first three units—*i.e.*, Puraka, Kumbhaka, and Rechaka is 1:4:2. This is rather drastic for non-professional Yogis. For beginners the advocated ratio is 1:2:1. They can gradually go on increasing the Kumbhaka in such a way that they will eventually need only about half the time for the Rechaka.

My advice to you is to keep the duration ratio of 1:2:1:1 for Puraka, Kumbhaka, Rechaka, and Shunyaka respectively, where 1 is anywhere between four and ten seconds, according to your capacity and convenience. Each breath should be slow, continuous, and deep.

16

Yogic breathing tones up and reconditions the intra-thoracic and intra-abdominal viscera (heart, lung, liver, stomach, colon, etc.), muscles, and lymphatic and blood vascular systems. Its effect on the nerves, the brain, and the mind as a tonic, sedative, and tranquillizer is remarkable. It substantially improves the longevity index. All these benefits have a very favourable bearing on the health of the spine.

Yoga and Diet

It is natural that you should want to keep physically and mentally fit. Correct diet is the main architect of the fitness of your mind and body. If your stomach is overfull or inflamed, if your bowels are unclean and full of poisons due to stasis and faulty peristalsis, not only will your body be sluggish but your brain, too, will be clouded and fuzzy. A clean and healthy bowel is a great asset to the health of the entire system including those viscera which are not directly connected with the processes of digestion and elimination. Simply taking care of your diet can attain this objective, rendering any medication utterly unnecessary.

Let the wholesomeness and health-giving nature rather than taste and decorative appearance of food decide your choice of it. If you observe correct habits—*i.e.*, if you do not eat too often or too much, you will be able to get away with a lapse now and then.

Starving yourself is not good for health even if it is done purposely in order to lose weight. You can achieve the same result, without starving, by a judicious combination of correct and nutritious diet and light Yogic exercises. It is not an exaggeration to say that correct diet and Yoga can make you feel healthier at eighty than you might have felt at eighteen.

Instinct and Appetite *v.* Tables and Charts

Nature had an infinitely earlier start in shaping and perfecting your appetite mechanism than the nutrition scientists had in preparing their food charts for you.

You already know that Yoga plays an important rôle in keeping the brain and the entire nervous system in a state of fitness and efficiency. Perhaps you were expecting me, in the present context, to talk of the stomach first, and not of the brain. But it is the

17

regulatory centres in the brain which control and direct the sensory system in your body to determine your food intake.

You are familiar with the food charts and tables that show the energy or calorie needs of various male and female age groups, and the amounts of proteins, carbohydrates, and fats supplied by various items of food, with their respective calorie values. These tables should be treated with respect, but are useful only to a degree. You can safely replace them by the remarkably precise yardsticks of your own instinct and appetite, which may prove even more reliable and more useful than the rigid figures of the charts.

This holds true of age-weight charts also. The tables prescribe the calories, the hours of sleep, the weights, the heights, and even the girths for different ages. Since there is no universally applicable standard, there is no need for the health-conscious individual to start brooding on the extent of his deviation from the norms detailed in the charts. Diet differs from individual to individual, from profession to profession, from circumstance to circumstance, and even from mood to mood.

The charts make no allowances for moods. A man in a state of anger or despondency may not feel like taking a single morsel of food. Regaling himself in congenial company, he may eat twice his normal quantity without having any awareness of over-eating or experiencing any physical discomfort. He may even digest it better than he would a small quantity consumed unwillingly, in a state of despondency.

The major articles of diet which supply energy to your body are carbohydrates, proteins, and fats. The calories made available to your body by these food components are:

carbohydrates	(1 gm)	4 calories
protein	(1 gm)	4 calories
fat	(1 gm)	9 calories

The daily calorie requirements of the moderately active average male, whose work is neither too light nor too heavy, are generally accepted as 3000 in U.K., 3200 in U.S.A., and 2800 in India. These three groups should, broadly speaking, represent most of the physical needs of the different peoples of the world. The calorie needs for women may be taken as 500 less than those required by men. The daily calorie needs in the case of men can come down to 1500 when they are off work and resting, and rise to 5000 for those who are doing extremely heavy work. They would be proportionately less in the case of women.

Both in Yoga and in Ayurveda, individualization is more important than generalization. Your reaction to food and associated factors, such as company, environment, etc., are your own; and your extraction of nutrition from the food you eat is also highly individual. That is why the instinct and appetite take precedence over the rigid and inflexible food chart when you are practising Yoga.

The essence of Yoga is non-dependence on external aids including food charts. The benefits to the body and the mind are achieved exclusively through the exploitation of their inner resources. Herein lies the chief merit of Yoga. Just as the means to liberate yourself from stiffness, aches and pains, anxiety neuroses, and morbid depressions and excitements, exist within yourself, so the means to regulate the food intake to your best advantage are in-built in your system.

A Warning

A modern doctor who read this discussion with much interest, and whose clinical acumen and skill—and professional and moral integrity—I consider of the highest order, has seriously questioned my wisdom in leaving you alone and unguarded with your instinct and appetite. He felt that I was taking a grave risk in giving you a free hand with your appetite. According to him, the prescribed Yogic approach might be all right for the disciplined people taking to Yoga earnestly. But, for the average Western man or woman, it might lead to indiscriminate and excessive eating.

This takes us back to the beginning of this book and the discussion under the heading "You and I", wherein I have referred to the bonds that existed between the teacher and the taught. So completely had I identified myself with you and your well-being, that the possibility of your abusing the trust I reposed in you in advising you to be guided by your natural appetite had never occurred to me until my attention was drawn to it by the doctor. I earnestly plead with you to heed this doctor's warning. However,

I am still inclined to trust you to discipline yourself and not betray the best interests of your health.

You are an intelligent adult. The fact that you are now reading this book is a proof that the will to improve yourself is already guiding your activities. You will find it easy to refine and control your appetite so as to make it the most reliable guide to your diet.

I therefore place the matter in your hands with the trust that you will belie the doctor's fears and fulfil my hope that you will achieve the improvement you desire not only in the shape of your body, but also in the discipline of your mind. The perfection of the physical figure is never more beautiful than when matched by the perfection of the mind.

Your Food

You are expending energy all the time, not only when you are working or thinking but even while you are resting or sleeping. A number of organs—such as the heart, lungs, kidneys, etc.—can never rest, and require a continuous supply of energy to maintain their activities. You have to spend energy in (a) promoting and maintaining the normal activities of the internal organs, (b) maintaining the body temperature, and (c) supporting the external physical activities of the body. You also need energy for (d) conversion of food into new chemical substances in the body. This energy comes from the food that you eat.

Yoga, through the centuries, has been closely associated with lacto-vegetarianism, with special emphasis on a non-stimulant vegetarian diet. Those of you who can take to purely lacto-vegetarian diet will find it rich in protein (milk, cheese, curd, nuts, soya beans, pulses, and many cereals and vegetables), in carbo-hydrates (cereal flours, rice, potatoes) and fats (butter, ghee, coconut oil, and other vegetable oils).

Those who cannot or do not wish to give up meat-eating, should try to confine themselves to lean meat, poultry, and fish, eaten sparingly twice, or at the most three times, a week. Even on these days, meat should be taken at only one meal. This is an ideal approach to diet while practising Yoga. It enables you to reap the maximum benefit out of your practice. However, it does not mean that if you are accustomed to eating meat in large quantities every day you cannot practise Yoga. Yoga will still benefit you but the

20

resulting gains will be smaller than if you are a lacto-vegetarian or as near one as you can manage to be.

The belief that vegetable sources supply only carbohydrates and fats and are deficient in proteins is highly erroneous. They are also excellent and vital sources of proteins, minerals, and vitamins, even when not supplemented with milk. With the addition of milk, the vegetable diet becomes an ideal nourishment, promoting not only vigour and efficiency, but longevity coupled with high physical endurance and tranquillity of the mind.

Daily Dietary Routine

Dinner is usually the heaviest meal of the day, and the whole night is given to its digestion. Breakfast and lunch are comparatively less heavy meals and one of these should be lighter than the other —*i.e.*, 60 per cent of your full meal.

Keeping the foregoing in mind, you may shape your diet on the following pattern:

1. BEFORE RISING
You can begin your morning with any of the drinks given below in order of preference:
Hot water, with 1 teaspoonful of fresh lemon juice (1 cup)
Hot water, with 1 teaspoonful of honey and 1 teaspoonful of fresh lemon juice (1 cup)
Fresh orange juice or fresh grapefruit juice at room temperature (1 to 2 cups)
Hot water only (1 to 2 cups)
Hot tea, with a teaspoonful of lemon juice (1 cup)
Hot tea, with 1 teaspoonful of honey, with or without 1 teaspoonful of lemon juice (1 cup)
Hot tea, with a dash of milk and sugar to taste.

If you are accustomed to drink a glass of plain water early in the morning soon after getting up, you can continue this excellent habit.

2. BREAKFAST
Vegetarians
Cereal: Choose your cereal and take it in any form you like. Butter or ghee (*i.e.*, clarified butter), honey, marmalade, jam, etc. Honey is preferable to marmalade or jam.

21

Fresh fruit or stewed fruit. Fresh or stewed fruit is preferable to tinned and preserved fruit.
Milk, buttermilk, or yogurt.

Non-vegetarians
Omelette, or boiled, poached, or scrambled egg; bacon, liver, or fish. Tea or coffee, with milk and sugar to taste, if desired.

3. LUNCH AND DINNER
Vegetarians
Soup (any vegetable).
Wholemeal bread (white bread for dyspeptics), well-cooked cereals, ground rice, or any other cereal preparations not fried and not containing much fat, with milk, cream, butter, cheese, cottage cheese, or honey.
Ghee, butter, or oil can be used for light application on chapaties and as a cooking medium.
Potatoes or sweet potatoes, dry-baked, steamed, or boiled.
Salad of raw vegetables.
Sweet dish—fruit salad, milk sweets, light milk puddings made with grated carrots, white gourd (Lagenaria vulgaris seringe) or white pumpkin (Benincasa cerifera, Savi).
Fresh fruit and nuts.
Finish with a cup of milk, skimmed milk, both preferably hot, or with buttermilk. This may be omitted.
If you feel thirsty, you can drink water with the meals. Those of you who do not drink at meal times should drink water half an hour or more later.
Tea and coffee are not desirable but are permitted if your urge for them is strong.

Non-vegetarians
Non-vegetarians can replace some of the food mentioned above by

Soup (meat or chicken)
Meat dish (meat, poultry, game)
Fish dish
Egg custard with fruit or sweet omelette.

Tea or coffee if desired.

4. AFTERNOON SNACKS

Vegetarians

Vegetable or cheese sandwiches, 1 or 2, preferably one. A piece of cake, or 2 to 4 biscuits. A cup of skimmed milk or weak tea or coffee with milk and sugar as desired.

Non-vegetarians

It would be better to have the same snack as vegetarians. If you are keen on a meat, egg, or fish sandwich at this time, omit the meat dish at your lunch.

Useful Hints

Always stop eating with the first feeling of fullness of stomach.

Take an apple, an orange, a banana, a biscuit, or a cup of fruit juice or skimmed milk if you feel uncomfortably hungry and the next meal hour is not near.

Develop a correct and healthy feel of the food requirements of your body. If you start putting on excess weight reduce the quantity of your food by 10 to 25 per cent. If you lose weight without intending to do so, raise the carbohydrate and fat content —*e.g.*, sugar, potatoes, bread, butter, etc., in your meals. If either complaint persists, do not hesitate to seek the advice of your doctor.

Alcoholic drinks are not conducive to the Yogic way of life and have therefore been omitted.

Spinal Pain

Pains arising out of injuries, infections like tuberculosis, and growths such as tumours, if involving the spine, require the attention of a specialist. You should not experiment with Yoga on these growths and lesions. But you need not suspend your deep breathing exercises unless some disease makes it too painful for you to expand your chest fully. However, since Yoga promotes tissue repair, and since tissue damage is believed to be a common effect of pain stimuli, it counters the tissue damage by making the nerves and the blood-vascular system healthier and more efficient.

The term 'spinal pain' or backache covers an unusually large number of different diseases ranging from cancer to ordinary fatigue, or even dislike for work, if you can call that a disease. It is certainly one of the commonest causes of pain. Persons of both sexes, of all ages from adolescence onwards, and from all walks of life get these pains which continue to harass them until either they change their profession or their attitude towards work. Yoga, whilst improving the tone of the aching tissues, contributes to the development of a mature attitude towards discharging one's duties.

When cancer or tuberculosis has eroded a part of the spine, Yoga, at the level you and I can practise it, cannot do anything to relieve the pain. Other conditions where Yoga cannot replace the specialist are dislocations, fractures, marked protrusion of intervertebral disc (mild slipped disc yields to Yogic exercises), pressure of malignancy on rectum or bladder causing reflex backache, and advanced curvatures of spine (scoliosis, kyphosis, and lordosis—i.e., lateral and antero-posterior bends). Under the guidance of an expert, some supplementary benefits can be derived from Yoga, and if the condition is mild and non-malignant, very considerable benefit is obtained from Yoga.

Before discussing the types of backache which respond favourably to Yoga therapy, I may also make a brief reference to certain conditions where the source of spinal pain lies outside the spinal area.

Colitis, dyspepsia, inflammatory conditions of appendix and gall bladder, gastric or duodenal ulcer, cardiac infarct, and abdominal malignancy, can cause referred pain in the lumbar spine in some individuals. Here, Yoga can prove a helpful adjunct to specific treatment of these conditions. It may even ameliorate some of these conditions—e.g., mucous colitis and dyspepsia, perhaps better than the medication itself, while being primarily resorted to to relieve the spinal pain. Invagination also is a cause of lumbar pain, peculiar to some women. This pain occurs when stools are obstructed by the invagination (infolding) of mucous membrane of the upper part of the rectum into the lower part. In the earlier stages, Yogic postures and Yogic breathing are helpful. Surgical intervention is required in later stages.

Women can also suffer from backache as a result of leucorrhoea, cervical ulcer, retroversion or prolapse of the uterus, inflammatory conditions of the internal urogenital organs, pelvic congestion, and

24

sexual dissatisfaction. These conditions all demand medical attention, but Yoga may also be helpful.

Inflammation of nerve endings (*e.g.*, peripheral neuritis) also lowers the threshold of pain. Yoga is helpful, but it is desirable to have the causal background checked and corrected.

Backache caused by fevers, such as malaria and influenza, is easy to diagnose and usually disappears along with the fevers, or soon afterwards.

Elderly people can suffer from backaches due to degenerative or inflammatory conditions of the bones (osteomalacia, osteitis, senile and post-menopausal osteoporosis, and osteoarthritis). Among these, osteoarthritis, particularly when not too advanced, even though very painful, is most responsive to Yoga therapy.

But you will find Yoga to be your best friend and greatest relief in the amelioration of the common backaches that form the main bulk of the complaint, namely the 'rheumatic' pains. These can be caused by chills, draughts, sudden exposure to cold after sweating, lifting a weight, sleeping in a cramped position, muscular strain, faulty postures, chronic fatigue, lowered exercise-tolerance, deformities imbalancing physical effort (*e.g.*, difference in length of legs), excessive use of back muscles (typing, writing, sewing, tailoring, gardening, horse-riding, sweeping and polishing floors, attending on children, etc.), and lumbar pains with negative laboratory findings revealing no known cause whatsoever.

Yoga and Sex

Your body has many limbs and organs which become progressively useless and atrophied through total and prolonged disuse. This does not apply to sex. The sexual faculty does not have to be exercised regularly in order to be kept in a state of normal efficiency.

However, it may be mentioned that the health of the spine and the nerves and other tissues associated with it has a considerable bearing on the health of the urogenital organs and on the sex impulse.

This book is on Yoga, which advocates celibacy; but Yoga is an associate of Ayurveda, which extends the definition of continence to include a life of moderation and which does not confine it, as some other disciplines do, to total celibacy.

Ayurvedic texts, while dealing with the symptoms arising out

25

of suppression of normal urges (*e.g.*, the urge to move the bowels, to sneeze, to sleep, to eat, etc.) have also mentioned the undesirable effects of undue suppression of the sex urge. This pragmatic view does not accept suppression of the sex urge as desirable. At the same time, it does not reject the higher Yogic objective—sublimation of the sex urge—and waxes eloquent on it. An Ayurvedic-cum-Yogic approach for the common man will favour a middle path, that of moderation. But moderation may be interpreted differently by different people; what is moderate for one person may be excessive or inadequate for another. The practice of Yoga has a remarkable effect in solving this problem efficiently and imperceptibly by levelling the excessive and the recessive urges to what may be considered a normal urge.

The contribution of Yoga to sex efficiency is very substantial. Through Yoga, the faculty is considerably renovated and toned up, and made to last much longer. Perhaps not many people are aware of the fact that if the mind and the body are normal, free from inhibitions, anxiety fears, and inferiority or guilt complexes, the sex desire neither 'weakens' nor turns into a mania or anything near it. More often than not, it is a psychic condition that keeps the mind continuously involved with sex. A healthy sex urge is like a healthy appetite—self-adjusting, appearing at the right intervals, and soothing and gratifying when appeased.

There is no better approach to sexual normality and efficiency than to leave it alone and let nature take its course. The formula is simple—if there is a genuine desire disturbing your mind and body, do not suppress it. If there is no desire, do not try to arouse it artificially.

The Asanas described here have been selected with the primary object of relieving you of spinal pain. But, as stated earlier, it is not possible to confine the benefits of Yoga to one particular organ. Almost every Asana contributes to the health and stability of a wide variety of tissues and organs. As such, these Asanas will naturally contribute towards the maintenance of a healthy sex impulse.

THE ASANAS

General Directions

1. Wake up before sunrise.
2. Avoid constipation. Train the bowels to move regularly by meticulous punctuality and the observance of a correct diet. Once Yoga takes over, you will automatically remain free of constipation.
3. Move your bowels before practising the Yogic exercises and breathing. Yoga is best practised on a clean bowel and an empty stomach.
4. You can take a hot or cold bath immediately before performing your exercises. A hot bath may be taken immediately after the exercises, but a cold bath should not be taken within 15 minutes of completion.
5. You can go through your exercises in the morning, taking 15–45 minutes according to the stage you have reached in your Asanas. Breakfast should be taken 30 minutes after completing the exercises, but if necessary this can be reduced to 5 minutes. You will find your body more flexible for exercises in the evening than in the morning. If it suits you better, you can take your exercise in the evening, provided you have not eaten anything for at least 3 hours preceding the commencement of the exercises. This is a compromise formula. Actually the Yogis demand a 4-hour abstinence from food preceding the exercises.
6. Prayers or meditation can be performed, if desired, while sitting in Sukhasana (Plate 1) or Padmasana (Plate 2), before or after you do your Pranayamic breathing exercises. If the prayer involves any ritual or a visit to a house of worship, let Yoga precede the prayer for better concentration.
7. Develop a habit of checking and re-checking your posture while standing or sitting, and go on correcting the faulty posture, again and again, day after day, until it becomes an unconscious habit with you to sit or stand erect without becoming stiff (Figs. 1 to 4).

27

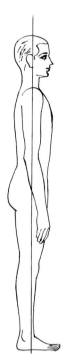

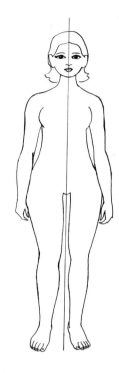

Fig. 1 Standing: Correct Posture   Fig. 2 Standing: Correct Posture

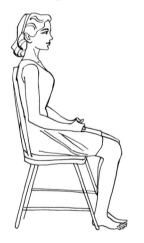

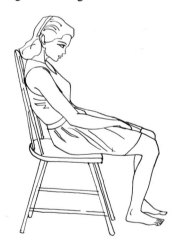

Fig. 3 Sitting: Correct Posture   Fig. 4 Sitting: Harmful Posture

28

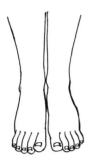

Fig. 5 Yogic Stance

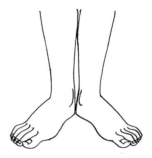

Fig. 6 Non-Yogic Stance

8. Relax your body with the following preliminary bending exercises before commencing the Yogic ones:

(*a*) Stand erect with both your feet joined together (Figs. 5 and 6).

(*b*) Stretch both your arms laterally, so that they make a straight line with both your shoulders (Fig. 7).

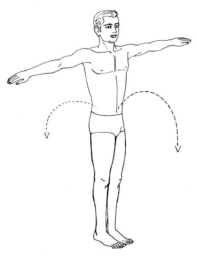

Fig. 7 Forward and Backward Bends

Slowly bend your body as far back as you can without torturing yourself or losing your balance. Having reached your limit in bending backwards, return to the original position as in Fig. 7. Then bend forward slowly, without bending the knees. Perform these bending exercises 3 to 5 times in each direction. (*c*) Raise your arms straight above your head attaining the maximum height you can (Fig. 8). Then, keeping your legs straight, bend forward, bringing down your arms to touch your toes (Fig. 9). Return to the original position as in Fig. 8. Repeat ten times. You can start with 5 bends raising the number to 25, if you so desire. 10 bends are quite adequate, normally.

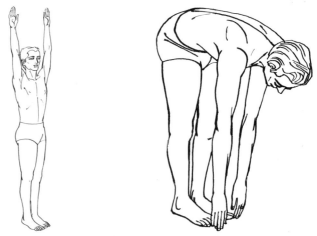

Fig. 8 Start of Touch-the-Feet Bends   Fig. 9 Finish of Touch-the-Feet Bends

9. *Important*. Exhale while bending, inhale while straightening your body to return to the normal position.
10. Lie down full length flat on your back (Fig. 10). Slowly lift both legs together, without bending the knees, till they are at right angles to your body (Fig. 11). Equally slowly lower them to the ground. Repeat ten times (Range: 5 to 20 times). Inhale while lowering the legs, exhale while raising them.

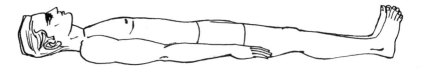

Fig. 10

11. Perform the exercises in the order given in the book, except that the Trikonasana (Plate 3) can be performed immediately after the preliminary bending exercises.
12. The time for each Asana should be half a minute for busy

30

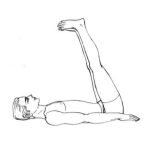

Fig. 11 Follow-up of Fig. 10

people. For the beginners, it can be a few seconds—*i.e.*, just as much as they can do without experiencing distress. Some discomfort, of course, has to be accepted in the earlier stages. 13. It is not necessary to perform all the Asanas. Choose those Asanas you are able to perform and stick to them, adding others as and when you can perform them equally comfortably.

14. *Important.* In case of backache caused by a slipped disc, omit those Asanas and preliminary exercises which require bending forward, and practise only those which require stretching the body and the spine backwards—*e.g.*, Bhujangasana (Plate 18), Matsyasana (Plate 15), etc., or such Asanas as do not require any bending at all, such as Vajrasana (Plates 10, 11), Gomukhasana (Plate 8), Matsyendrasana (Plates 5 to 7), etc. Dhanurasana—*i.e.*, the Bow Pose (Plate 19), is an exception, and should be avoided.

15. Perform the Pranayama—*i.e.*, the 4-unit breaths described on page 92 twenty-five times, after completing your Yogic postures. The last pose—*i.e.*, the Shavasana or the Pose of Tranquillity (Plate 32) is performed last of all, after the Yogic breathing exercises.

16. **The Yogic exercises described in this book are designed to prevent spinal pain. If, however, your back is already giving you pain, you should consult your doctor before starting these exercises.**

31

1. Sukhasana — Easy Pose

Posture: Sit on the ground with the legs folded at the knees so that both the heels are touching your body with one foot resting inside the knee-fold and the other beneath it as shown in the picture.

This posture is widely practised by laymen in India at the time of meditation, worship, and prayer. It is easy to perform and a good substitute for Padmasana (Lotus Pose). Those who cannot perform Padmasana in the earlier stages can use Sukhasana until they can sit comfortably in the Lotus Pose. All Yogic breathing or postures with which Padmasana or Lotus Pose is prescribed as the basic posture can be practised with the help of Sukhasana (Easy Pose) by those who find it difficult to sit in the Lotus Pose.

Benefits: The main benefit of this posture is its availability to beginners as a vehicle for Pranayama (Yogic breathing exercises). It eliminates exhaustion and fatigue after strenuous games, drills, or heavy manual labour. Next to Shavasana (Pose of Tranquillity) and Vajrasana (Hardy Pose) this is the best pose for relaxing the muscles of the body, including those related to the spine.

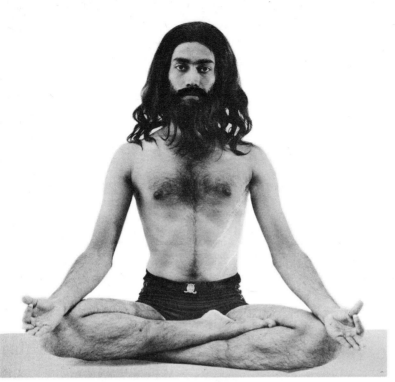

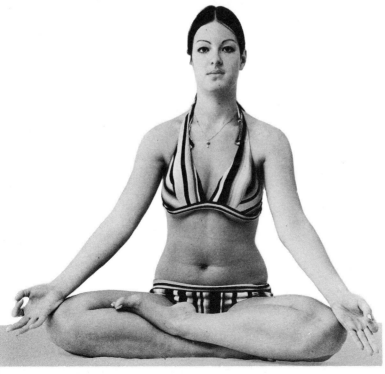

2.   Padmasana — Lotus Pose

Posture: So called because the soles of both feet are turned up and the feet diverge like the petals of a lotus flower. Sit down on the ground with your legs and feet loosely resting in front of you. Stretch the left leg at right angles to your body with the heel resting on the ground, then hold your right foot by the ankle and bring it up to your left groin placing it on the left thigh with the heel so close to the body that it presses against the groin. Without disturbing the position of the right foot, flex your left knee so that the left foot comes near the body. Lift it from the ankle and place it on your right thigh with the heel of the left foot pressing against the right groin. Straighten your spine with the chest slightly pushed down in the front. Place your two hands on your knees as shown in the photograph.

This is the best pose for Pranayama—*i.e.*, the exercises for cultivation of control of breathing. Those who are too obese to complete this pose can just put their right foot on their left thigh for three minutes and then change over and place the left foot on the right thigh for three minutes. This should be continued till the practice develops sufficiently to enable you to perform the Lotus Pose.

Benefits: This posture bestows all the benefits of the Easy Pose (Sukhasana) shown in Plate 1. It is considered superior to Sukhasana as the benefits are more pronounced. The Yogis attribute to this posture the capacity to activate the spinal cord, and to improve the Yogic breathing and its effectiveness. The practice of Yogic breathing while sitting in this posture keeps the spinal column straight and firm. It contributes to the tranquillity of the mind and is, therefore, recommended as the ideal posture for meditation, concentration, and study.

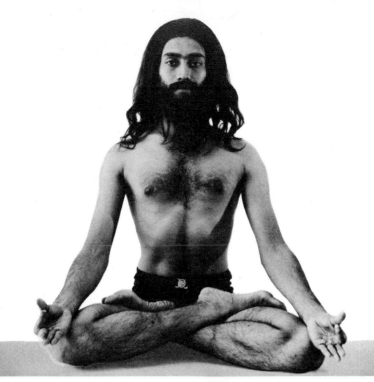

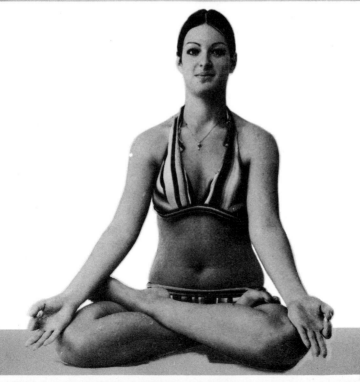

3. Trikonasana — Triangle Pose

Posture: Stand erect with both feet wide apart, stretch your arms on both sides keeping them parallel to the ground, then keeping the arms firmly in position start bending on your right side till your trunk is parallel to the ground and your right arm is touching your right foot. Your two arms at this stage make a straight line at right angles to the ground. Make sure that you bend only laterally. Fight the tendency to bend forward while attempting to bend in the lateral plane. A variant of this pose is to lower the left arm gradually towards your head, without bending it in the least, till the arm also is held in the horizontal plane touching the left side of your head and held parallel to the ground. Keep your eyes open and continue deep breathing. Repeat the posture on the left side.

Benefits: The main purpose of this Asana is to dissolve the 'spare tyre' around the waist. This is one of the few postures stretching the waist in the lateral plane on both sides. It will be observed that the bending in most of the postures is either forward or backward. This posture therefore covers areas affected only partially by the other postures. It imparts an all-round flexibility to the body. It streamlines the figure by slimming the waist and developing the lateral muscles of the hips, thereby giving shape and grace to the hip line.

This is a favourite posture for women, who can safely perform it even during the first six months of pregnancy. The Yogis claim that it improves the functioning of the lungs, purifies the blood, removes rashes, boils, and pimples, and imparts glow to the skin of the body in general and the complexion of the face in particular. There should be no jerky movements when performing the Asana. All movements should be slow and graceful.

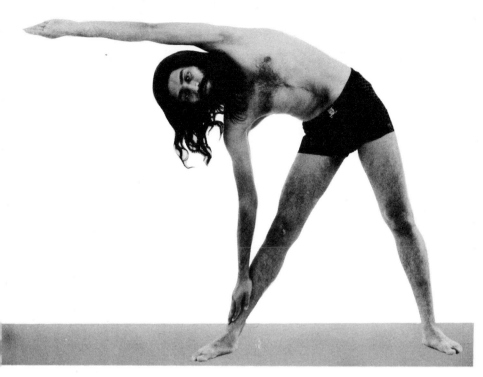
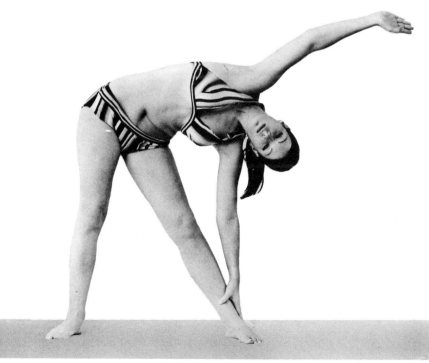

4. Utkatasana — Squatting Pose

Posture: Stand on your toes with the heels raised as high as possible. Then slowly sit down on your heels without lowering them to the ground. The entire weight of the body remains on the toes. Your thighs and calves, joined together, should make a parallel line with the ground. The rest of your body should be erect and at right angles to the ground. Place both hands on your knees. Keep the eyes open. Continue deep breathing.

Benefits: This posture improves the tone of the muscles of toes and ankles in particular and of the legs and feet in general. Yogis attach considerable importance to this Asana as a basic pose for performance of some cleansing processes in Yoga style, such as Jalavasti (water douche) and Pavan-avasti (air douche) for emptying the intestines. It is also considered to be a promoter of continence by acting as a sedative on the sex centres. In addition it helps in developing a correct posture for the spine.

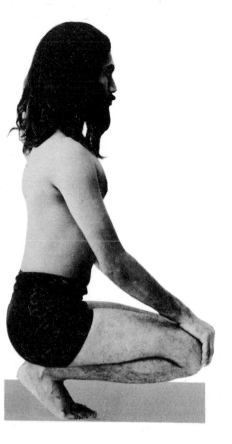

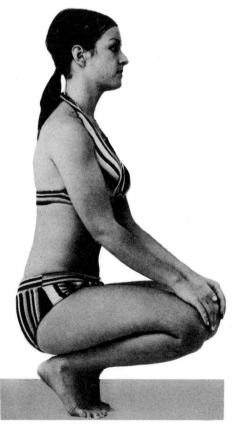

5. Ardha Matsyendrasana — Incomplete Matsyendra Pose I

Posture: Matsyendra was the name of a great ancient Indian Yogi. He used to sit in this posture which is named after him as Matsyendrasana. Ardha, in Sanskrit, means 'half'. Here, the name of the posture is preceded by half (incomplete) as the beginner will find it difficult to perform the complete posture.

To perform the incomplete posture, sit on the ground and spread the right leg in front of you at right angles to your trunk. Then place the left foot on the ground on the right side of your right knee as shown in the plate. Then pass your right arm around the left knee and hold your foot with your right hand. Take your left hand behind your back placing the back of your left hand on the extreme right of your waist. Continue deep breathing and expand your chest as far as possible. Turn the head to your left as far as it can go and tilt the turned head downwards so that the chin touches the left shoulder. Keep the eyes open. Do not let the knee of the right leg rise from the ground. Try to press your abdomen with the upper part of your left leg while in this position.

Repeat the same in reverse by stretching the left leg and putting the right foot beside the left knee, and so on.

Benefits: This posture is usually prescribed for people with weak kidneys and lax urinary (bladder) muscles. It alleviates spermatorrhoea in the case of men and leucorrhoea in the case of women. Leucorrhic discharge resulting from serious lesions like cancer, abscesses, or venereal infections would, of course, need medical treatment under expert guidance. The practice of this Asana bestows many other gains which are described among the benefits of the complete Matsyendrasana (Plate 7).

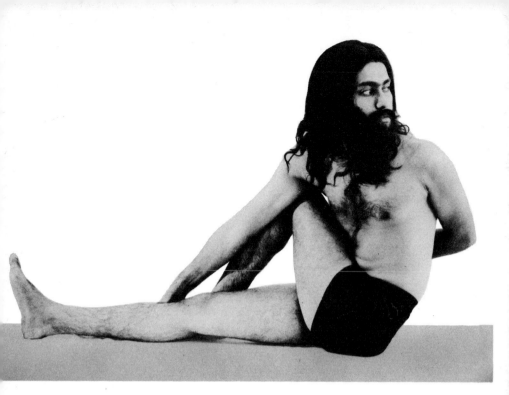

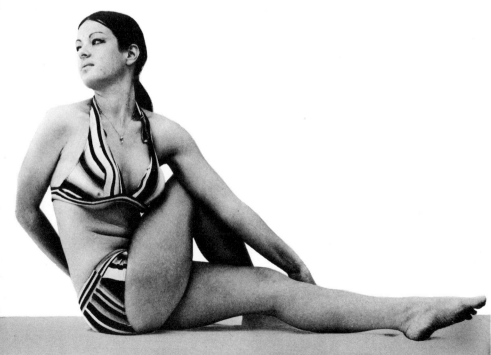

6. Ardha Matsyendrasana — Incomplete Matsyendra Pose 2

Posture: The same as in Plate 5 except that the stretched leg is drawn in so that the heel touches the opposite hip.

Benefits: The same as from the previous Pose.

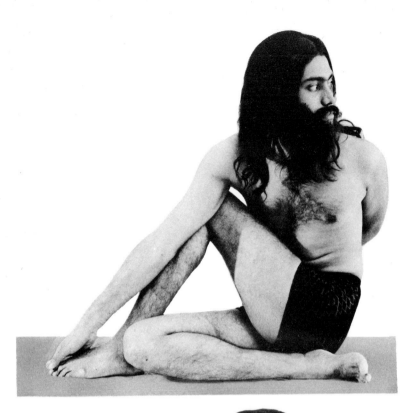

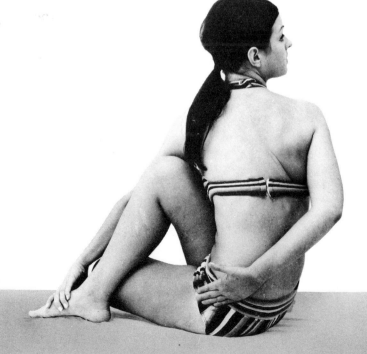

7. Purna Matsyendrasana — Complete Matsyendra Pose

Posture: Sit on the ground and place the left foot on the right thigh as you do in the Lotus Pose. The heel of the left foot is near the navel. Now raise your right foot and place it beside the left knee as you did in the previous incomplete posture 1, the difference being that here the right leg is not stretched. See that the entire sole of your right foot by the side of the left knee is touching the ground and does not leave it. Then bring your left arm around the right knee and catch hold of the toes of the right foot with your left hand exactly as you did in the reverse pose in the Incomplete Matsyendra Asana 2. In the same manner take your right arm behind your back and bring it to a position so that it touches the left heel, instead of just the waist as in the former posture. Turn the head to the left, touching the left shoulder with the chin.

Repeat the Asana in reverse placing the right foot on the left thigh and changing the position of the limbs in the preceding posture.

Benefits: This posture compresses the alimentary canal and almost all the viscera lying in the thorax, the abdomen, and the pelvis. It also twists the spine alternately on both sides and stretches the muscles of the legs and the arms. When fully accomplished, the Matsyendra posture hardly leaves any portion of the body unexercised and unstimulated. Yogis prescribe it for the disorders of the liver and the spleen, particularly when they become chronic. It is very beneficial in chronic backache, toning up the nerves and the deep as well as the superficial muscles of the spine. It improves the blood circulation of the entire body, increasing the efficiency of the spine in particular. Apart from spinal pain, it alleviates the pains in various parts of the body served by spinal nerves as it adjusts and corrects the malpositions of the vertebrae

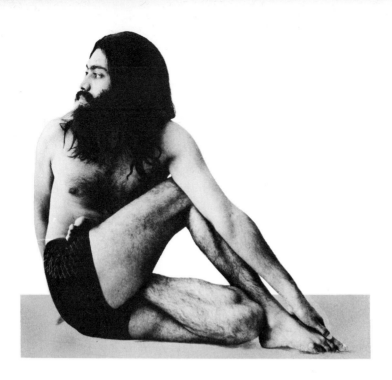

and even the deformities of the spine in general. By maintaining deep breathing during this pose, the exerciser accelerates the blood circulation of all the glands and viscera from thyroid down to the pelvis including the sex glands. It also improves digestion and assimilation of food and alleviates dyspepsia. Some Yogis go as far as to attribute anthelmintic properties to this posture—*i.e.*, destruction of worms found in the alimentary canal. How far it is effective in killing and expelling the worms is not possible for me to corroborate but there is no doubt that the practice of Matsyendra Asana is very beneficial to the exerciser in search of sound health and longevity. It is a difficult pose and only through long practice and patience can average men and women master it. It is for this particular reason that I have offered a compromise in the form of the Incomplete Matsyendra Asana, to enable the reader to gain some if not all the benefits of this posture.

8. Gomukhasana — Cow-Head Pose (Front View)

Posture: Sit on the ground with the right leg bent so that the centre of the rim of your heel is under the anus. The left leg should also be bent so that the left heel is as much under the right hip as possible. Sitting in this posture take your right hand behind your back so that the elbow bend is in contact with your head. Then take your left hand behind your back keeping the left elbow under your left shoulder. Then lock both your hands together behind your back as shown in Plate 9. The front aspect of the posture is shown in Plate 8. Keep the eyes open, body straight, and abdomen slightly contracted. Continue slow and deep breathing.

Benefits: This posture improves the circulation in the armpits and the sides. It also tones up the tissues of the feet, the knees, and the waist. It improves the circulation and tones up the muscles, tendons, and ligaments of the knees and the calves. The practice of this Asana, alternating the position of the two arms, improves the circulation and activity of both the lungs. It has been recommended to those suffering from tuberculosis of the lungs. It is beneficial to patients of asthma and also tends to disperse axillary glands. It is very helpful in relieving backache. It removes feelings of weakness and fatigue and of dislike for food. It also tends to reduce hyperacidity (heartburn).

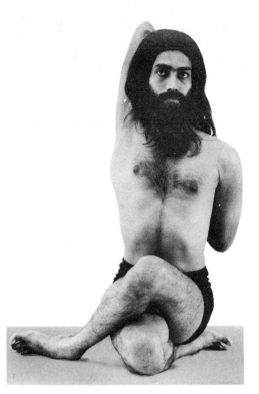

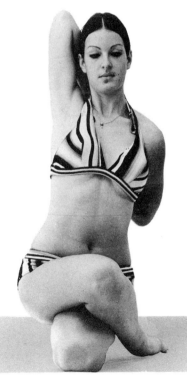

9. Gomukhasana — Cow-Head Pose (Back View)

For description of this posture and benefits read page 46.

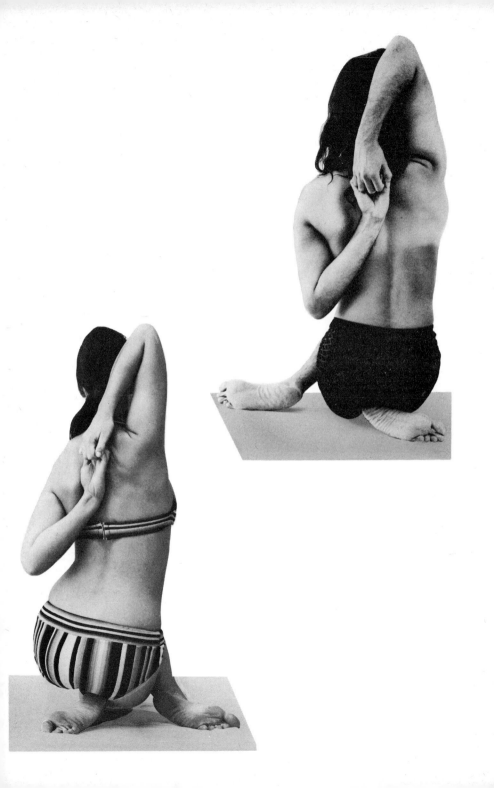

10. Vajrasana — Hardy Pose

Posture: Kneel on the ground with the knees, ankles, and big toes together. Then slowly sit down on your heels, still keeping the heels and the big toes together. Put both your hands on your knees as shown in Plate 10. Keep the chest expanded and abdomen drawn inwards. The head, back, and waist should be kept in a straight line. Keep the eyes open. Take deep breaths. Do not tense the body, but relax and feel comfortable.

Benefits: This posture is particularly good for those whose backache is aggravated after a heavy meal. It should be practised immediately after meals by persons with a history of heart disease who experience discomfort after their main meals, particularly in the epigastrium (pit of the stomach), and who sometimes get palpitation due to pressure of gas on the diaphragm. It helps digestion. Heart cases with dyspepsia are advised to practise this posture for five to ten minutes after breakfast, lunch, and dinner.

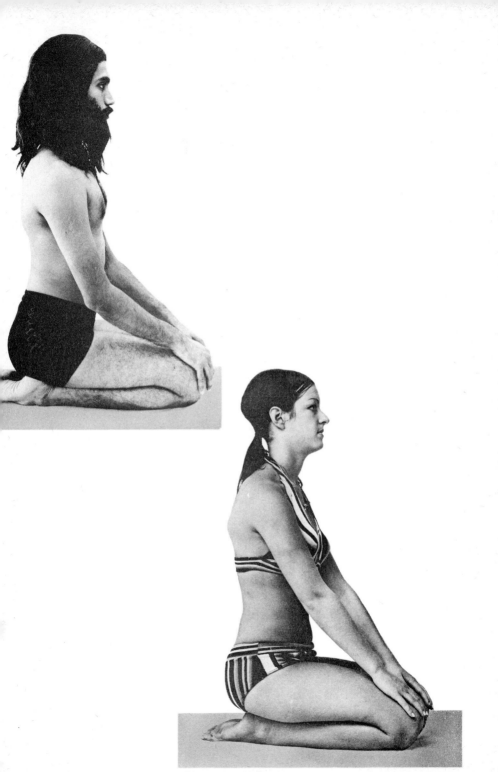

11. Supta Vajrasana — Horizontal Hardy Pose I

Posture: First place yourself in the posture preceding this one—Vajrasana (Hardy Pose). Then, raising your back with the help of your hands, stretch your head as far back as you can so that your back is arched above the ground while the entire body rests on the head at one end and the lower part of the legs and feet at the other. Keep both your hands on your thighs. Continue deep breathing. Pregnant women should avoid this pose.

Benefits: It exercises the muscles and the blood vessels of the feet, knees, abdomen, ribs, thorax, throat and neck, mouth, eyes, and the head, and benefits all these parts. The exerciser experiences a stretching sensation the whole length of the body. In spite of this feeling you should keep your body and mind as much relaxed as you can. This exercise corrects certain defects of the spine, alleviates backache, and tones up both the deep and the superficial muscles of the spine.

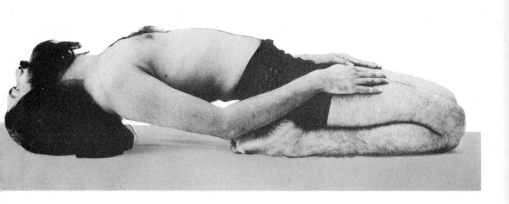

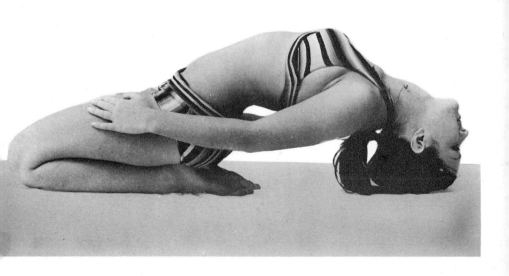

12. Supta Vajrasana — Horizontal Hardy Pose 2

Posture: Kneel on the ground with the knees, ankles, and big toes together. Then slowly sit down on your heels, still keeping the toes together. Without shifting the position of the toes and the knees and only just separating the heels to make a place for your seat, bend slowly backwards till your head and shoulders touch the ground behind you. Keep both your hands on your thighs. The entire back also should be as much in contact with the ground as possible. The eyes can be kept open or closed. Continue deep breathing. Remain as much relaxed as possible during the posture.

Benefits: As described for the previous posture.

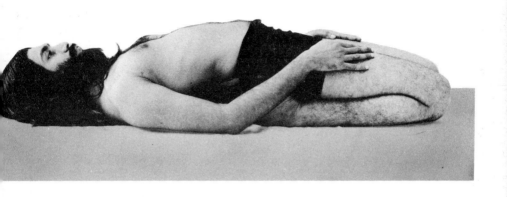

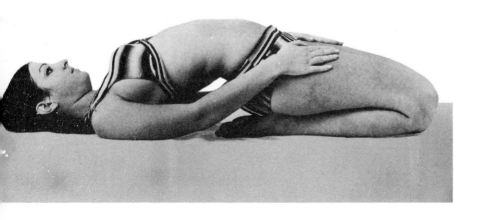

13. Urdhwa Sarvangasana — Shoulder Stand Pose

Posture: Lie on your back full length, legs together and arms touching your sides. Raise your legs and trunk so that the entire weight of the raised legs and trunk is borne by the shoulders. The elbows should be resting on the ground with both hands and the forearms supporting the back to keep the body erect and in position for the posture (See Plate 13). From the tip of the toes down to the shoulders the entire body should be in a vertical straight line at right angles to the ground. The chin should be pressing against the lower part of the neck. The elbows should neither be too far from the body nor too near it. Try to flex the feet and the toes upwards as much as possible. Do not bend the knees and keep still though relaxed. Fix your gaze on your toes. If this results in the eyes watering, close them and relax. Breathing during this posture should continue to be deep and slow.

It may not be possible for obese people to perform this Asana to perfection. Probably they will be able to raise only their legs and not the trunk. This should not discourage them. They should raise their legs as far as they can without feeling much discomfort and distress.

Benefits: The Shoulder Stand improves the circulation and the neuromuscular tone of the eyes and the brain. It also improves the functioning of the throat vessels and vocal chords and improves the voice of singers. Experiments have confirmed that it improves the functioning of the liver, improves digestion, and tones the nerves and musculature of all the communication channels linking the head and the trunk. It is a prophylactic against many diseases. Yogis attach great importance to this posture as an aid to awakening of the Kundalini, the mysterious power capable of leading the Sadhaka (Aspirant) to Absolute Perfection. However, you and I, the normal inhabitants of this world, also stand to gain much benefit from this excellent posture, which is equally

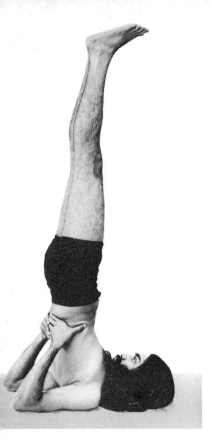

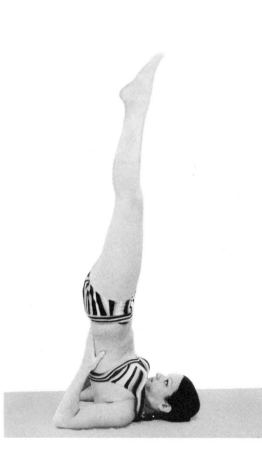

good for men and women alike, conferring practically all the benefits that the headstand (Shirsana) bestows, without resulting in any of the harmful effects which the latter sometimes entails.

14. Halasana — Plough Pose

Posture: Lie down on the ground on your back, raise the legs upwards, then raise the back with the help of both hands until you attain the Urdhwa Sarvangasana (Shoulder Stand— Plate 13). Then tilt your legs slowly until your toes touch the ground behind your head. Keep your legs straight and do not bend the knees. Then stretch your arms behind your back so that they rest in the opposite direction to the legs. The arms should rest on the ground parallel to each other with the palms touching the ground. The body now rests on the shoulders, neck, and head. This pose resembles a plough and is therefore named after that implement. Keep the eyes open. If you cannot continue deep breathing in this posture, you can breathe normally while holding this pose.

Benefits: This Asana is also known as Sarvangasana which literally means 'all-parts posture'. It exercises and stretches the posterior muscles of the entire body. It improves the circulation and tone of the whole length of the spinal cord, and at the same time benefits the arms and legs. It tones up the thyroid gland. It imparts elasticity and pliability to the spinal cord, 'oiling' the roots of the bilateral nerve branches of the spinal cord (32 pairs in all, serving the major part of the body). The stretching involved in this exercise enlarges the passages (vertebral foramina) through which the branches of the spinal cord pass out into the body, thereby raising considerably—and sometimes spectacularly—the efficiency and performance of the entire spinal nervous system and the areas served by it. Its regular practice improves the functioning of the thoracic and abdominal viscera in general. It improves the circulation of the brain thereby contributing to intelligence, alertness, and good memory.

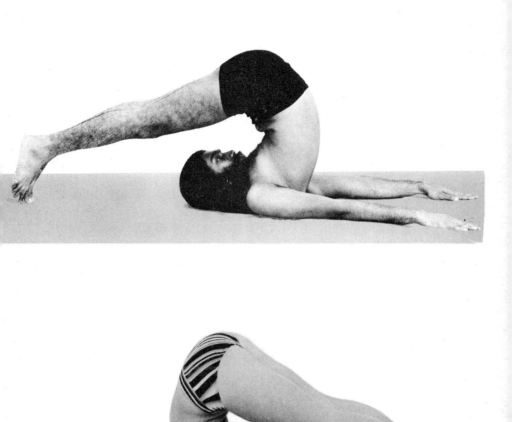

15. Matsyasana — Crocodile Pose

Posture: First, sit in the Lotus Pose (Padmasana), then gradually bend backwards until you are lying on your back with the legs still fixed in the Lotus posture. Flex your head backwards and arch your back by raising your chest and abdomen so that the entire body rests on the knees and the head. The head should be stretched backwards so that the highest point of the head is resting on the ground. Breathe slowly and deeply, feeling relaxed.

Benefits: This posture relieves constipation and tones up all the tissues of the spinal column. It is said to be particularly beneficial to women as it normalizes uterine functioning.

It tones up the lungs and muscles of the chest. It improves the circulation of the throat and tends to reduce tonsils. It is said that those who practise this posture regularly maintain a strong and erect spine even during old age. Even if one has developed a slight stoop, regular practice of this posture will help to correct it. It is also said to help diabetics by improving their general metabolism. People suffering from spinal pain should practise it regularly. There is no harm in practising it in part if you are unable to achieve the perfect posture. Even while practising an imperfect posture, the exerciser should keep his mind and body free from tension and rigidity. If it is not possible to eliminate tension completely it should be reduced to the minimum.

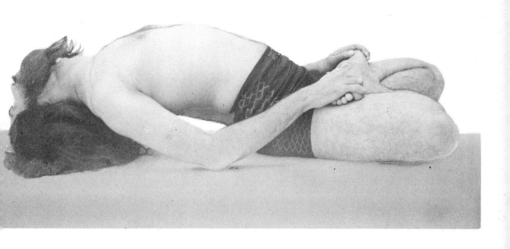

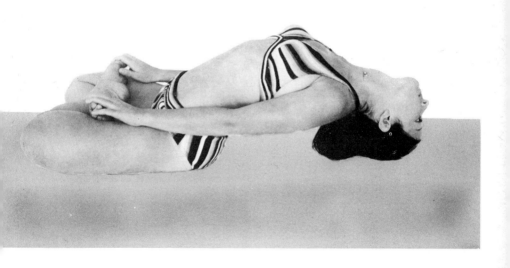

16. Ushtrasana — Camel Pose

Posture: Kneel down with only your knees and toes touching the ground. The heels should be raised so that the soles are at right angles to the ground. Then stretch your head backwards in an effort to touch the base of the neck with your head. Bend your waist backwards so as to enable your hands to hold your raised heels without bending the arms. In this pose your chin (pointing skywards), ears, and heels should be in a straight line at right angles to the ground (Plate 16). The eyes can be kept closed or open. The entire body should be firmly held in position without becoming tense. Deep breathing should continue. After you get tired fill the lungs with air and sit down slowly on your calves. Terminate the posture after a few deep breaths in this position.

Benefits: This posture improves the tone and circulation of the deep and the superficial muscles of the spine from the neck down to the coccyx, or tailbone. Some Yogis claim that it is very beneficial in cases of fistula and piles. It alleviates constipation and reduces rectal inflammations (if they are not malignant).

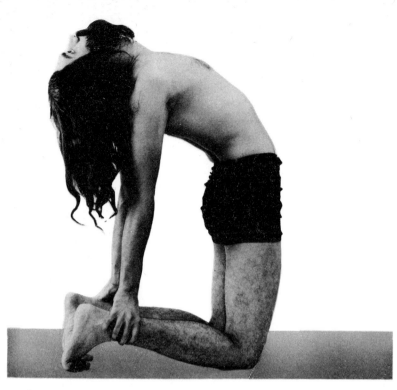

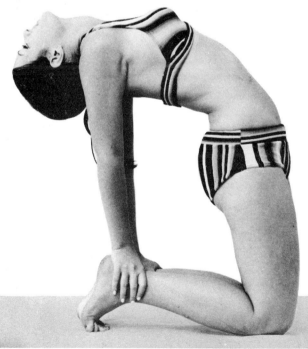

17. Pashchimottanasana — Posterior Stretch Pose

Posture: Sit on the ground with your legs stretched straight in front of you so that the body is at right angles to the legs. Then stretch your arms in front of you so that the arms are parallel to the ground. Start bending forwards and lower the stretched arms so that your hands touch your toes. Now start bending your trunk forwards and downwards till your forehead touches the legs. In the perfect posture the head rests on the knees and the index fingers of both the hands are hooked round the toes while the elbows of both the arms bend slightly inwards and even touch the ground on both sides (see Plate 17). Keep the eyes open, breathe normally. Keep in this position for some time, then return to the original position—*i.e.*, forming a right angle between the legs and the trunk with the hands resting on the knees or the thighs, and relax.

Beginners might find it difficult to attain this posture to perfection during their earlier efforts. This should not discourage them from practising it, for, even when it is imperfectly performed, the benefits to be obtained from it are many.

Benefits: This posture stretches the spine to its maximum length. Therefore its contribution to circulation, and to the tone of the spine, spinal muscles, and spinal nerves is considerable. It reduces abdominal obesity, removes stiffness from the posterior muscles and imparts elasticity and flexibility to the lower back. It alleviates muscular pains especially in the lumbar and dorsal regions and the legs. Some Yogis advocate this posture for controlling repeated hiccups and asthmatic attacks. Its benefits to general health are considerable.

Take special care to perform this movement rhythmically; exhale while bending forward and inhale when returning to the upright position.

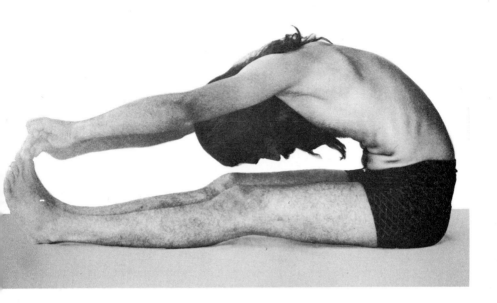

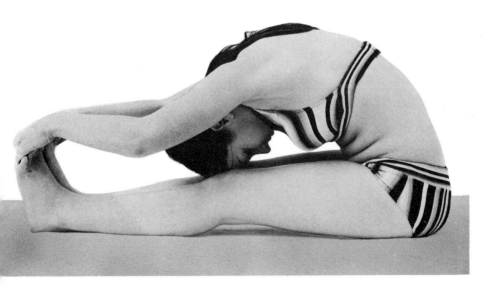

18. Bhujangasana — Serpent Pose

Posture: Lie down full length on your chest and abdomen; then, placing both your hands on the ground alongside your shoulders, raise your chest on your arms as high as you can with your head stretched backwards. The body from the waist down to the toes should remain in touch with the ground, the legs and the feet being held together. Breathe slowly and deeply.

Benefits: This is an excellent pose for reducing abdominal fat and relieving constipation and flatulence. Its contribution to relief from spinal pain is remarkable considering the simplicity of the pose. If practised patiently and diligently it helps the exerciser to get over spinal pain of long standing, even when caused by osteo-arthritic changes in the spine. Its benefits affect the entire length of the vertebral column, including the cervical, the thoracic, the dorsal, and the sacral vertebrae, and the coccyx (these words denote the divisions of the spine into the neck, the upper back, the middle back, the lower back, and the tailbone respectively). It also tones up the muscles, tendons, and ligaments, the nerves and the blood vessels of the spinal region.

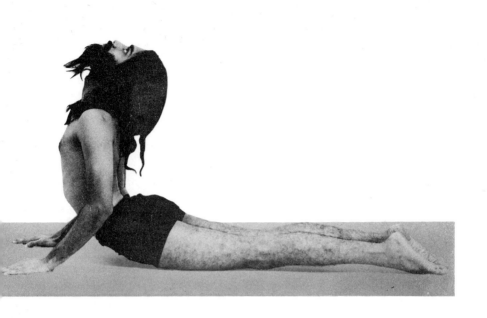

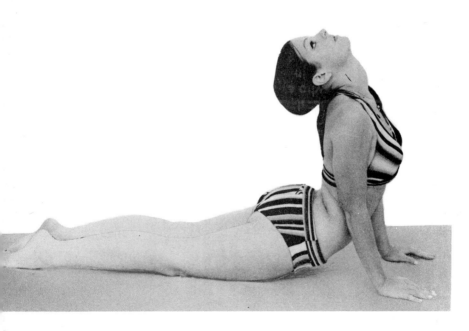

19. Dhanurasana — Bow Pose

Posture: Lie down on your chest and abdomen with your arms resting alongside your body. Throughout the exercise both the legs and the feet should remain joined together. Lift both the feet and legs upwards and backwards, bringing them towards your head until, with your arms raised behind you, you can hold both the ankles, the left ankle in the left hand and the right ankle in the right hand. The head should be held high. The chest also should be raised from the ground so that only the abdomen and the pelvis remain in contact with the ground. The pose should be held steady without any movement except that of the respiratory tract. Fill the lungs with air before raising the legs and the chest. At the completion of the pose continue normal breathing if deep breathing appears to be difficult. The feet may tend to come down towards the waist, but if you remain firm in your pose you can hold them steady. Keep the eyes open. Fill the lungs when returning to the ground to terminate the pose.

When you are accustomed to this posture learn to rock backwards and forwards (like a rocking chair).

Benefits: This posture, too, exercises the entire body. It strengthens the deeper and the superficial muscles of the entire spine, removing rigidities, stiffness, aches, pains, burning sensations, and tenderness of the spine and areas adjacent to it and served by the branches of the spinal cord. It tones up and develops the muscles of the chest. It improves the function of the liver, the kidneys, the bladder, the genital organs, and other pelvic and abdominal viscera. It is a prophylactic against the formation of stones in the kidney and gall bladder. It relieves scanty, painful, and burning urination. Practised regularly in middle age, it has a healthy effect on the prostate and protects against enlargement or inflammation of this gland. It gives relief against piles, anorexia (dislike for food), flatulence, and halitosis (bad breath) when not caused by pyorrhoea. This Asana should not be done by those suffering from slipped disc.

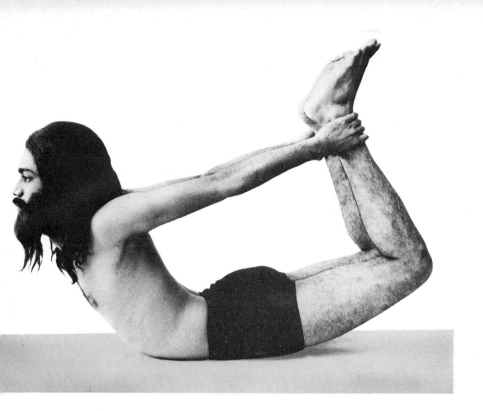

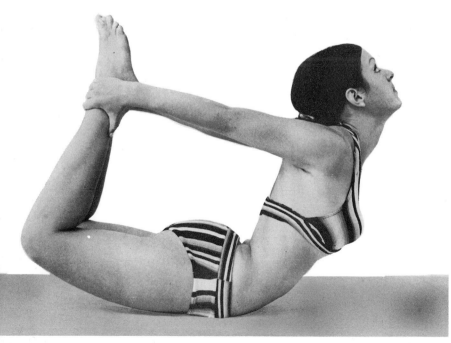

20. Eka-Pada Shalabhasana — Locust Pose I

Posture: Lie down straight and full length on your abdomen with both your arms close to your body remaining on the ground. The chin also should be touching the ground. The upper surface of the stretched feet should also be in contact with the ground. Then take a deep breath and raise the left leg as far above the ground as you can without experiencing too much difficulty or distress. Then slowly exhale and take five deep breaths. Again fill your lungs with a deep breath and slowly bring down the leg into the original position. Repeat the entire process with the right leg. During the exercise do not bend your knees and do not take the leg out of its straight line with the body.

Benefits: The Locust Pose streamlines and dissolves fat from the knees, hips, waist, and abdomen. It tones up the muscles of the dorsal and sacral spine. It counters tendencies to constipation and piles. It improves the circulation of the lower intestines and removes flatulence. It also removes the aches and pains of the areas referred to above. Yoga teachers particularly recommend this posture for practice by women.

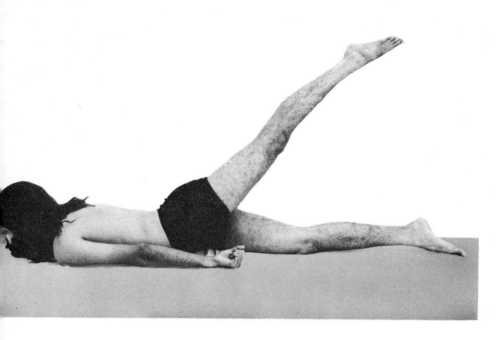

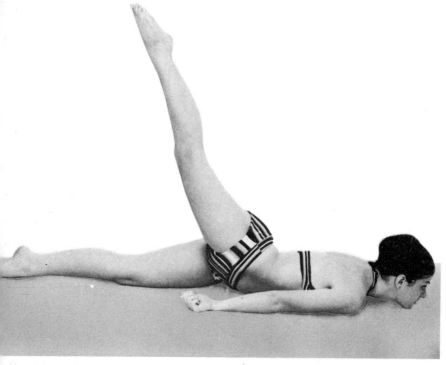

21. Dvipada Shalabhasana — Locust Pose 2

Posture: Lie down on the ground, face downwards as in Pose 1 described on page 70. In both postures 1 and 2 the arms and hands should be on the ground, the entire length of the arm touching the body right up to the sides of the thighs. Fill the lungs with a deep breath, raise both the legs upwards as far as you can take them without experiencing too much discomfort or distress. Take three to five deep breaths in that position. Again fill the lungs with a deep breath and slowly bring the legs down till they rest on the ground. Do not bend the knees and throughout the exercise keep both the legs straight; the legs should not separate. The chin should remain in touch with the ground. The exerciser will not be able to raise the legs very far from the ground. Only through long practice will the requisite flexibility to practise the posture efficiently be acquired.

Benefits: This posture tones up the ligaments, tendons, muscles, and nerves of the lower back and the waist in general. It improves the circulation of the entire pelvic region, toning up all the organs and viscera of the area. It is said to tone up the urogenital apparatus. It reduces oedema of the ankles and feet. It is good for women suffering from dysmenorrhoea and irregular menses. In addition it is also helpful in relieving piles and early stages of fistula. Yoga teachers also prescribe this Asana to patients for painful urination, diabetes, and scanty urine as an aid to the treatment they may be undergoing.

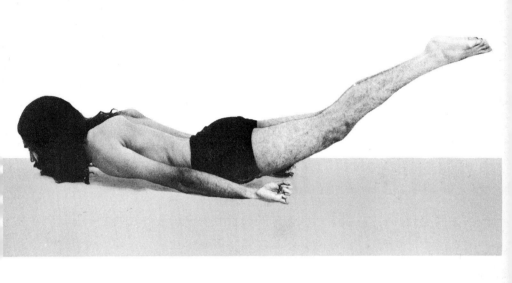

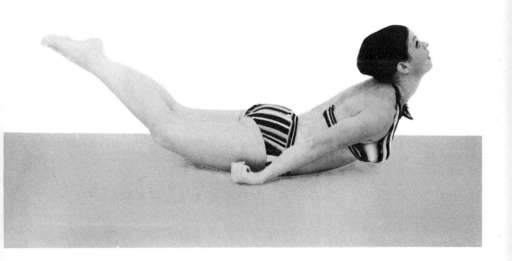

22. Naukasana — Canoe Pose

Posture: Lie down full length on your chest and abdomen with your arms behind your back. Do not bend your elbows and lock the fingers of both the hands together. Then fill the lungs with a deep breath and raise your head and chest and the legs as far above the ground as you can without experiencing discomfort or distress. The body should be held thus resembling a canoe. The entire weight of the body should be borne by the abdomen.

Benefits: This posture improves appetite, stops hiccups and excess of eructations (belching). It expels gas. It improves the functioning of the digestive system including that of stomach, liver, duodenum, and small and large intestines. It ameliorates 'phlegmatic' disorders including colds and catarrhs. It tends to lessen the force of asthma attacks and de-aggravates fistula. It tones up the muscles of the chest and dissolves abdominal fat.

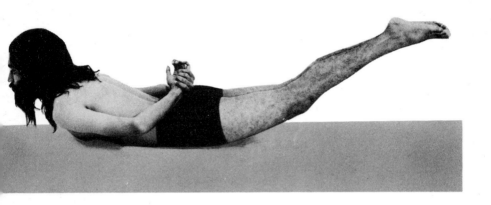

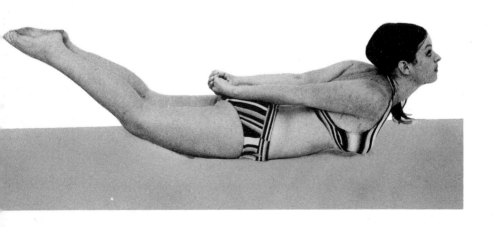

23. Supta Urdhwa Hastasana — Raised Hands Pose I — Lying Down

Posture: Lie down on the ground on your back with your hands placed behind your head and arms stretched to their maximum length. The length from the tips of the fingers to the tips of the toes should be increased to the maximum possible by stretching the entire body including the arms and legs as if the extremes of the body were being subjected to a pull in opposite directions. Even the neck should be stretched as far back towards the hands as possible.

Benefits: This posture confers the benefits of traction on the spine and the rest of the frame. It relaxes and improves the functioning of the neuro-muscular structures. It also improves circulation.

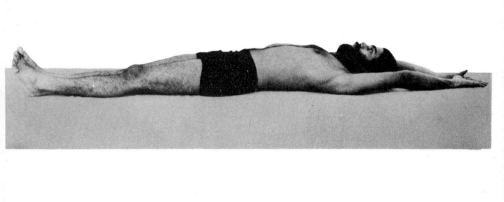

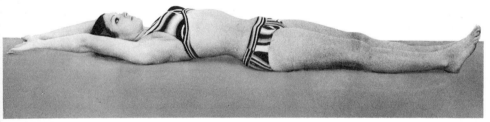

24. Supta Urdhwa Hastasana — Raised Hands Pose 2

Posture: From the lying down posture described on the preceding page raise yourself slowly into the sitting position without disturbing the position of the raised arms which should move upwards in an arc remaining in a straight line with the body. The posture is completed when the trunk of the body is at right angles to the stretched legs which remain in the original position. From this position bend forward, again in an arc, keeping the raised hands in the same position in relation to the rest of the body. The bending forward should continue till the hands touch the toes. Those unable to bend so much as to be able to touch the feet should bend forward as far as they can, and from that position start bending backwards again till the back and the arms touch the ground and the exerciser reaches the position described in the raised hands posture 1 (preceding page). In this Asana the exerciser should slowly exhale while rising from the ground and bending forward and inhale when bending backward. In other words one should breathe out when folding the body and breathe in when unfolding the body.

Benefits: This posture along with the exercise that accompanies it strengthens the muscles and the ligaments of the spine, particularly the dorsal and the sacral spine, and prevents tendency to sciatica, the pain that travels from the hip joint downwards to the back of the knee or even further affecting the whole leg down to the heel. It also tones up the abdominal muscles and improves the circulation of the organs of the digestive system. It alleviates chronic constipation and improves appetite. It dissolves the extra fat of the abdominal wall.

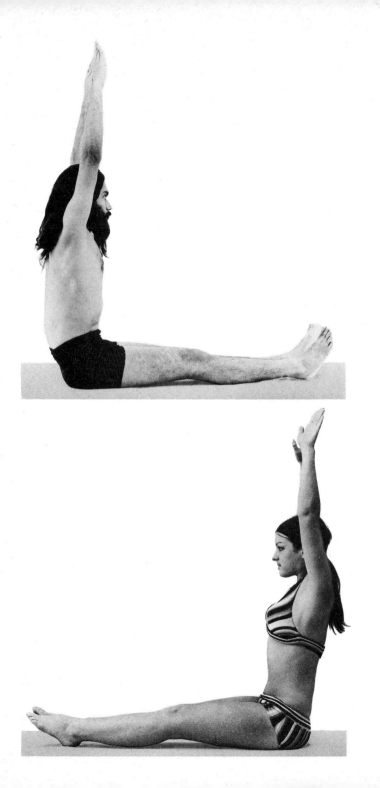

25. Chakrasana — Wheel Pose

Posture: Lie down on your back. Draw up the knees so that the heel of each foot touches the corresponding hip with the soles of the feet resting on the ground. Place your hands one on each side of your head with the elbows pointing upwards and the palms and the fingers resting squarely on the ground. Then supporting the weight of your body on your hands and feet raise your hips and abdomen as high as you can so that the entire body describes an arch with only the hands and the feet touching the ground (Plate 25). Keep the body as still as possible. The hands and feet should hold the ground and remain firmly in position. Raise the back as far up as possible so that the body imitates the shape of the rim of a wheel as much as possible. Fill the lungs with air before raising the body. Continue deep breathing during the posture. Fill the lungs again with air before slowly returning to the ground at the end of the exercise. After lying down on the ground deep breathing should continue for a few seconds. The eyes may be open or closed.

Benefits: This posture keeps the spine young and flexible even during old age. It helps the exerciser to retain the flexibility and lightness of all the dorsal and ventral muscles. The Yogis prescribe this posture for improving the eye-sight, and the richness and clarity of the voice. It is also claimed that it tones up the lymph glands and clears inflammatory conditions. It improves the texture and the complexion of the skin. It also gives relief in cases of constipation, flatulence, nausea, and asthma. It removes unpleasant sensations (pins and needles, burning, tenderness, pricking, general debility, rigidity, and anorexia, or lack of appetite). It tones up the nerves serving the organs of sight, hearing, smell, and taste. It also improves the circulation of blood to the brain thereby contributing to intelligence and alertness.

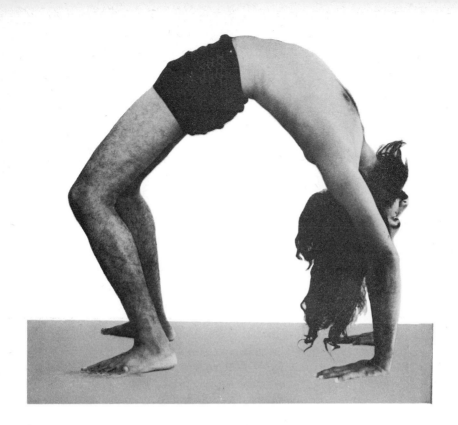

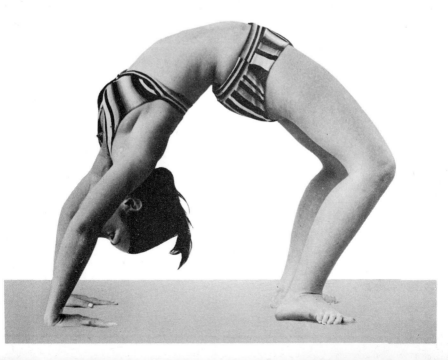

26. Vrikshasana — Tree Pose

Posture: Stand erect on the ground, raise your arms above your head, the tips of the stretched thumbs of the hands joined together. Now raise your heels keeping your entire weight on the toes. Pull and stretch the whole body towards the sky as high as possible. Hold yourself firmly in this pose, keep the eyes open, and continue deep breathing. At the termination of the exercise lower the heels slowly to the ground and also release the arms to let them come to your sides.

Benefits: This exercise has the effect of mild traction on the spine. It also tones the toes and the soles of the feet by stretching the muscles and improving the circulation. The Yogis also recommend the use of this exercise for nervousness, debility, and pains and aches in the chest and sides. It is thought that if the exercise is started early it can help young children and adolescents to increase their height.

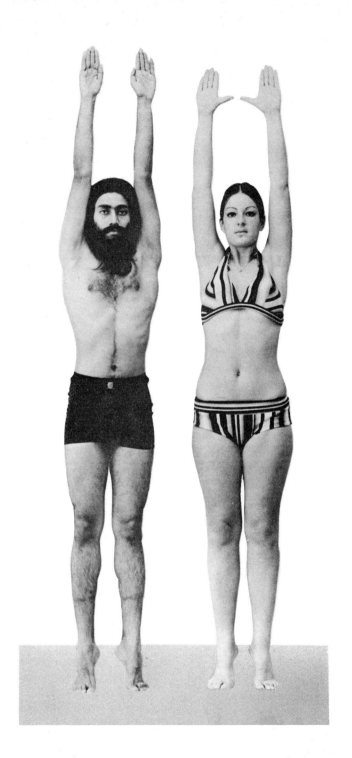

27. Mayuriasana — Peacock Pose

Posture: Kneel on the ground keeping your knees apart, so that the palms of both your hands touch the ground in the centre of the space between your two knees. Then bend forward keeping the palms of both the hands on the ground and bringing together the two elbows so that both the elbows afford a support to your abdomen. Then, balancing the weight of the body on the forearms as the palms remain on the ground and the elbows take the weight of the body, throw back the legs and the knees so that the length of the entire body is now parallel to the ground but resting above it on the elbows so that the palms of the hand are the only parts of the body in contact with the ground. While in this position, draw in the legs crossing the forelegs in the way of the Lotus Pose (Padmasana, which is shown in Plate 2).

This is a very difficult pose and takes time to cultivate. It is the only posture (apart from Purna Matsyendrasana) which Miss Herman has not been able to demonstrate correctly (see plate opposite).

Benefits: The practice of this posture coupled with correct, light, and healthy diet improves the functioning of all the abdominal organs of digestion and elimination—e.g., liver, spleen, kidneys, stomach, intestines, and bladder.

An M.D. attached to one of the biggest hospitals in Bombay has trained himself to practise it, as it is his experience that it has helped him to get rid of "a chronic annoying pain in the ribs and backbone".

This posture is not recommended for cases of diarrhoea, dysentery, high blood pressure, epilepsy, diseases of the eye, bronchitis, and fainting fits. It is considered particularly good for women with a weak and lax uterus and men with weak reproductive tissues.

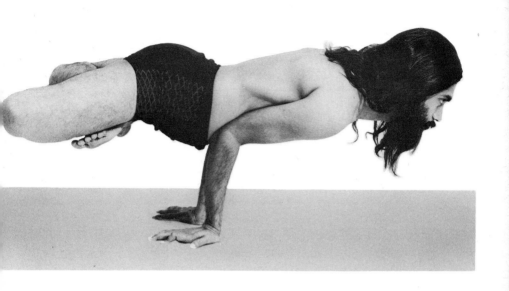
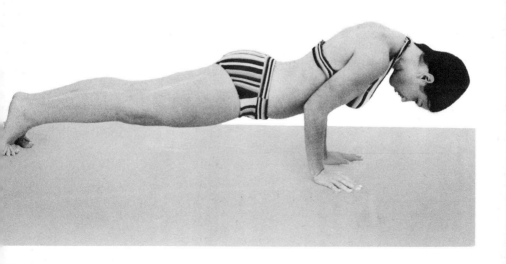

28. Surya Namaskara — Obeisance to Sun Poses 1, 2 and 3

Surya Namaskara is a special set of connected exercises constituting the ancient Indian salutation to the sun after the morning ablutions and bath. I have selected only three postures from the series—each has a bearing on spinal pain.

Posture 1: Stand facing the rising sun. Raise your arms keeping them in a straight line with the body, hold them firmly in that position and keep the legs straight, without bending the knees. Bend the entire body above the waist as far back as possible. Inhale deeply while bending backwards (see Plate 28). Continue to breathe deeply. To terminate the posture fill the lungs with a deep breath and slowly return to the standing position. Keep the eyes open but perform the exercise before the sunlight gets strong enough to dazzle the eyes.

Posture 2: Squat on your left foot, stretching the entire length of the right leg backwards. Place both your hands palm downwards on the ground. Keep your arms straight and do not bend the elbows. Keep the heel of the left foot raised from the ground so that it is in contact with your left hip. Flex your head backwards as far as you can take it. Remain steady in this pose keeping your eyes open and taking slow and deep breaths (see Plate 29). Take a deep breath, bring the right leg forward placing the right foot alongside the left and terminate the pose. Reverse the posture.

Posture 3: First sit in posture 2 described above. Then lift both the hands from the ground, raise them high above your head without bending the elbows. The rest of the posture beneath the waist should remain exactly in the position shown in the second posture. Bend the body above the knees backwards stretching it as far back as possible keeping the arms in a straight line with the trunk (see Plate 30). Slow and deep breathing should continue. Straighten the body with a deep breath and terminate the pose as in posture 2.

Benefits: Great religious and spiritual significance is attached to Surya Namaskara due to its age-long association with the worship of the morning sun. The three postures described here help to cure aches and pains in the spinal area and neutralize the deleterious effects of the prolonged bending which labourers, housewives, typists, clerks, etc. are forced to undergo. Surya Namaskara dissolves the adipose tissue not only of the abdomen and the back but also of all other parts of the body benefiting practically all tissues of the body including nerves, tendons, ligaments, muscles, blood vessels, and various glands and viscera of the system. The convention lays down that the Surya Namaskara should be performed in the mornings only, just as the sun is rising.

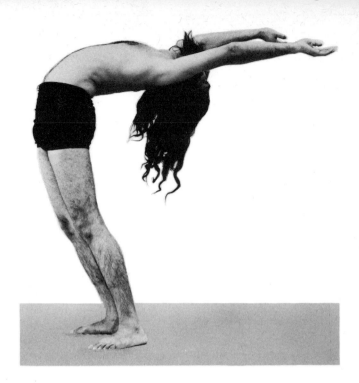

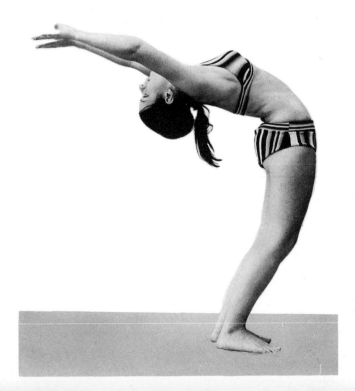

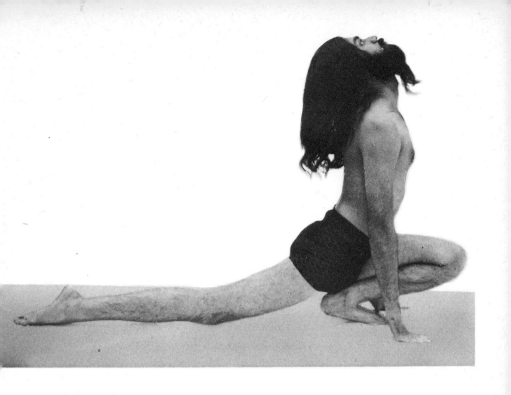
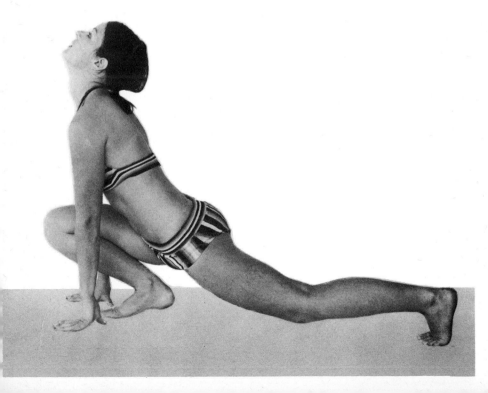

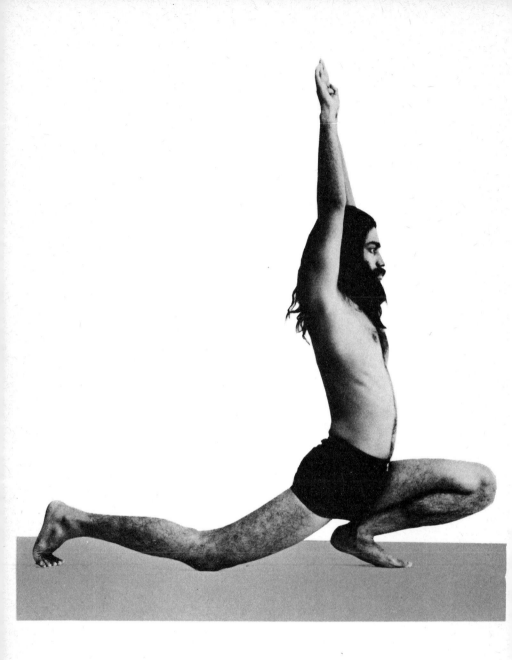